Please remember
    as you go through life
to take these special
        things with you--
the knowledge
        that you're capable,
the faith to make
        your dreams real,
    the feeling that
        you're truly
        a person
            of worth...

SANDCASTLES
on the FARM—

Fighting for Hope

JEAN HADSELL-HAHN RUSCO

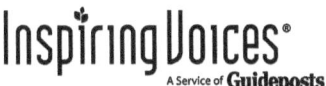
InspiringVoices®
A Service of **Guideposts**

Inspiring Voices books may be ordered through booksellers or by contacting:
Inspiring Voices
1663 Liberty Drive
Bloomington, IN 47403
www.inspiringvoices.com
1-(866) 697-5313

All scripture references were taken from the Woman's Devotional Bible and the New International Versions of the Bible.

Any people depicted in stock imagery provided by Thinkstock are models, and such images are being used for illustrative purposes only.

Certain stock imagery © Thinkstock.

Scriptures taken from the Holy Bible, New International Version®, NIV®. Copyright © 1973, 1978, 1984, 2011 by Biblica, Inc.™ Used by permission of Zondervan. All rights reserved worldwide. www.zondervan.com The "NIV" and "New International Version" are trademarks registered in the United States Patent and Trademark Office by Biblica, Inc.™

Scripture taken from Woman's Devotional Bible.

Most names have been changed to protect the providers and other persons.

ISBN: 978-1-4624-0439-1 (sc)
ISBN: 978-1-4624-0440-7 (e)
Library of Congress Control Number: 2012922426

Printed in the United States of America

Inspiring Voices rev. date: 01/29/2013

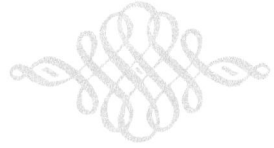

Dedication

THIS BOOK IS DEDICATED to my three children; Paul, Lisa, and Malee. Their encouragement and support during my cancer and follow-up physician visits and subsequent complications with lens replacement surgeries kept me positive for my future life existence.

This book carries a special dedication to our infant son, Saul Erin, who was torn from us at birth.

Also, special credit goes to my five grandchildren--Dawn, Cooper, Erin Breann, Jacob, and Will. Their presence in my life has granted me the courage to fight cancer so that I may live to enjoy more time with them.

As cancer survivors say, "live for more birthdays".

And most of all, praise and dedication I give to the Heavenly Father for holding my hands and carrying me through this crisis. He definitely left footprints in the sand.

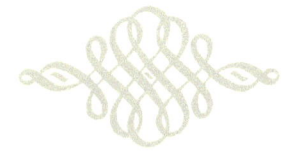

Introduction

MY MISSION IN WRITING this book and sharing my experiences as a cancer survivor is to offer insight to others who are interested in head or neck cancer or who have been diagnosed with this type of tumor. Also, to show the cancer survivor's life experience could be used as research or insight into other's who have some form of head or neck cancer.

My desire is to provide more information to promote donations for Head and Neck cancer research. Currently no government funds are available for this research, as this type of cancer is so rare.

My goal is to prove that faith can bring you through to be a survivor.

Words I live by...

"But those who hope in the Lord will renew their strength. They will soar on wings like eagles; they will run and not grow weary, they will walk and not be faint." –*Isaiah 40:31, Woman's Devotional Bible, New International Version*

CHAPTER I

Embracing Shock

IT LOOKED LIKE WE were driving on a highway through a deep gorge. A blizzard a week ago had dumped seventeen inches of snow with fierce blowing winds to create deep drifts. Being in labor with a baby, my husband was driving us to the small hospital during the cold frozen night. I was only experiencing intermittent contractions of the lower back; going on for a good twelve hours. The snow plow had made huge piles of snow on each side of the black highway which gave an eerie feeling of almost being in a tunnel. As we approached a main intersection, I stated to him:

"Turn here, let's go to Great Bend. Take me to Central Kansas Medical Center" (a larger regional hospital).

He replied, "You have to trust your doctor."

The viewing and graveside services for baby Saul Erin went on without me. I was still hospitalized. My husband had to do all the final arrangements. The infant loss of my baby boy has greatly impacted my life. The sorrow was tremendous and always reappears at the death of another loved one in my life.

Christian singer, Natalie Grant, has a top of the charts song called "Held," and it is so fitting. She sings about life taken away and empty arms. After losing my only brother to ALS, Lou Gehrig's disease, at age fifty-five, then losing my father and 5 years later, my mother, that song brings the grief back every time.

At a follow-up appointment with my doctor after outpatient surgery in a Day Surgery Center to remove polyps in my nose, he examined my nasal passages and told me they were healing well. But his next statement hung upon me as grief.

"I don't have very good news as far as the lab report goes," he said, pausing a moment before continuing. "I will do the best I can for you; the report from pathology is that you have a tumor in your nose called an sarcoma," He paused again, "all sarcoma are malignant."

Shock set in, and I protested, "My ex-husband is diabetic; my firstborn was stillborn. This can't be!"

I sat there, stunned and numb. Then I stuttered, "But—It's not fair, losing a full term baby; losing my brother to ALS; lost my parents recently—; and now this!"

Dr. Dinswald, the ear, nose, and throat specialist (ENT), took my hand and said emphatically, "I'll get you to the best place for treatment. I took my training at Dallas Medical Center, and doctors on staff there are my friends. I can set you up for visits and testing immediately. Or, I can refer you to Dr. T. Grant, ENT, at Kansas University Medical Center (KUMC) in Kansas City. Either of these places can give you a second opinion. I'll get you to the best facility for treatment." He was so caring; like I was a family member. I know he felt awful having to tell me.

Dr. Dinswald walked me to the reception desk and asked the office assistant to set up an appointment with Dr. T. Grant at Kansas

University as soon as possible. He turned to me and said it would take about fifteen minutes to make the arrangements.

Trying hard to hold on to my composure, I told him I needed to make some phone calls and that I would wait in my car.

"That's fine," he said.

As I closed the office door and stepped out into the hallway, the tears crept into my eyes. I walked down the stairs and out the door as quickly as I could, almost running. I then sat down in the driver's seat of my car, trying to make sense of everything that had just happened. The sobbing continued for several minutes. Then my thoughts drifted to an earlier time…

CHAPTER II

Harvest as a Farm Wife

THE BLUSTERY WIND KICKED up a swirl of dust from the sandy road. As I close the window on the truck, I run my tongue over my teeth to remove the gritty feeling in my mouth.

I smile as I watch both combines crawl through the golden wheat field like huge crabs; they chop off the wheat heads and beat them against the rolling paddles. Chaff spills out the back of the machines and rotates in the air, creating a tiny whirlwind. My truck comes to a slow, rolling halt after I carefully guide it through the field "get-in" (drive in). I pedal on down the beaten path to the end of the field, where the combines will stop to unload their precious cargos of grain.

This harvest time is an adventure anticipated all year—a cure for the stresses that drought, flood, gale, early or late frost, harsh winter, and dreaded hailstorms create for both farmer and crop. One of Mother Nature's only mercies is snow cover—snow cover is good for the crop, as it keeps harsh winter winds from drying the roots.

As the day ends, all crews shut down between 11:00 p.m. and 12:00 p.m. At this point, the grain draws moisture and is too wet to cut. Grain growers' crops have to meet an acceptable moisture content reading in order for the grain elevators to accept the loads of grain.

Back at the house, I strip the bandana from my head. It had been tied tightly around my hair to keep it free of the blowing dust and itchy wheat chaff; it also kept the flying strands of hair out of my eyes. My face appears like a painted mime—not white, but dark with the dirt covering my skin. I say to myself, *"probably breathed in that much dusty dirt, too"*. I slosh my face with cool, clean water and watch the dirty liquid spill into the sink. *"There is so much of it,"* saying to myself again. I blow my nose to get as much dirt out as I can. I clear my throat again, as I did many times today, to dislodge the dirt and chaff collected there. My thoughts drift, *"seems that during harvest we always have hot wind to go with it"*. But the dust and wind is part of living in Kansas, so I dismiss it from my mind and think of it no more.

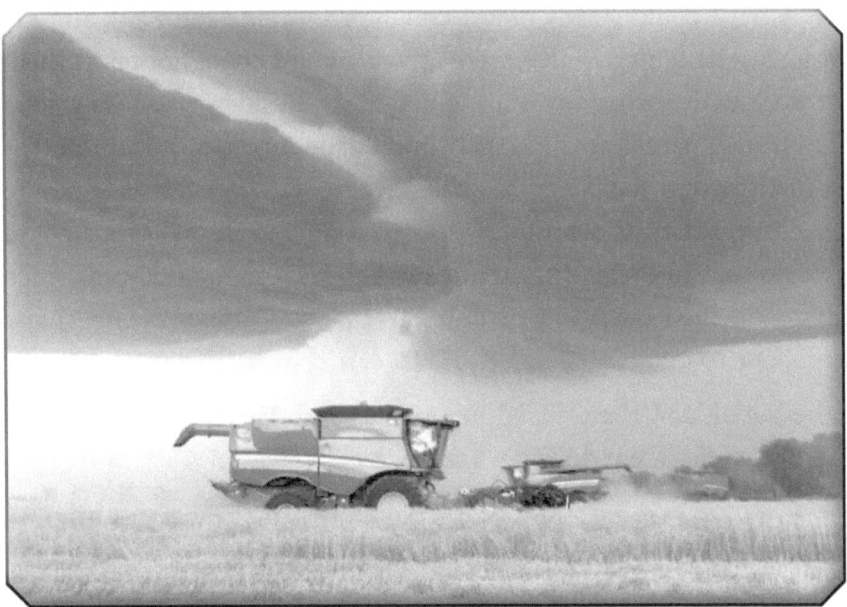

Typical picture of wheat harvest, combines working as fast as possible because an impending storm that approaches.

CHAPTER III

Back to Reality

Now, still sitting in my car, I wanted to call my children, but I couldn't. My oldest daughter Lisa, my son Paul, and my youngest daughter, Malee, were at work, and I could not upset them at work with such a devastating diagnosis. Besides, when they get a call from a parent at work, their immediate reaction is to think that something has happened to their diabetic father; such as, a severe insulin reaction to warrant hospitalization and near death. I could not do that to them. They'd already had such numerous calls since living on their own. I just wanted to talk to a family member; just someone to talk too!

I hesitated, and then dialed my ex-husband. He answered as usual with a gruff, "What do you want?"

"For God's sake," I said, "can't you ever answer pleasantly?" I immediately broke down and started crying.

He paused, letting me cry for a moment, and then softly asked, "What's wrong?"

"I have cancer," I sobbed.

"Where are your doctors?" he asked.

I answered, "My doctor, from the Lawrence Otolaryngology Group, is sending me to Kansas University Medical Center in Kansas City for a second opinion."

"Don't worry," he reassured me. "It sounds like you are in good hands."

"I'm scared. I don't want to do more surgeries or see any more doctors!"

"Wait to see what KU says," he said, patiently reassuring me again. We hung up, and I put my face in my hands and cried for some time.

When I finally looked up, the nurse was flagging me from the clinic door. I returned to the office and met with the appointment clerk. She had set the date of my appointment for a week away with Dr. T. Grant—the ear, nose, and throat specialist at Kansas University Medical Center—as May 25, I had to wait six more days.

But when I returned to my car with my appointment papers, my thoughts drifted back again to my first years on the farm, and my soul felt uplifted. I thought of my kids' cheerful bedrooms, the crackling warmth of the fireplace, and what fun it had been to decorate the house with real pine and cedar evergreens. The smells clearly came to mind. *Will I be able to smell again when all of this is over?* I wondered. *Will I even live through it?*

Here I am parked under the shade of a big pine tree. I had the window down and could smell the scent of pine. I sobbed for some time, wishing so badly that I still had my mother here on earth—but she'd been gone for two years. I so wanted to spill everything to her. It would have made me feel so much better, and I know she would just hold me, hurting with me.

I called my sister, Lea, and told her my cancer situation. She asked me several questions, what kind of cancer? How are they going to treat it? Where are you going for care? After answering her questions, we talked a few more minutes. She asked that I keep her posted about details.

The office visit with Dr. Dinswald flashed through my mind, again as I replayed the details of his words. I could hear him say, again, when I was in the exam room, "Everything looks good. I was able to remove some of the polyps in your nose."

He hesitated, then turned away to grab a sheet of paper sitting on the cabinet top. He picked it up and turned back to me, saying slowly, "Although...the lab report is not good news."

In reminiscing that fateful, horrifying scene again, I listen carefully to his next words.

"There is a cancerous tumor in your nose, and we're not sure if it is in all your sinus cavities and growing behind the right eye. We do know the CT scan shows it about one-sixteenth of an inch from the brain lining."

I heard him say, "I'll send you to the best place there is." Then he took my hand. "Let's start with an appointment with the Kansas University ENT doctor for a second opinion."

This was May 19, 2010. I slowly drove to my apartment. I called my work supervisor and said I would not be in for the rest of the day. Next, I called my friend Patti, but she said she was sick and couldn't talk.

"Patti!" I yelled, "Did you hear what I just said? I yelled, "I have cancer!" She again said that she was sick. I hung up, feeling disgusted and angry. All I could think about was how many times I'd been there for her when she'd experienced two job losses and estrangement with her daughter. It was such a hurting feeling that she did not care enough about me; as I so badly needed to talk to only friends and family.

Then the anger set in.

"Why me, God? I lost a baby. I had an ill husband for years—a Type I brittle diabetic. I have worked since my youngest, was three and a

half years old. I had to return to college to acquire a degree so I could support my children. Finally, I had to go through a divorce, because my husband was not taking care of himself and us. And now, cancer? I wanted to scream!"

It didn't seem just. Only two years prior, I had inherited a small amount of money from my parents. I'd wanted to re-establish my home, restore my marriage, as my ex-husband was finally taking care of himself regarding his diabetic condition. I just wanted to put my life in some kind of order. Now I wasn't sure if any of that was going to happen.

I pulled my daily notebook from my basket of special things kept by my easy chair. I always wrote down special things to remember in this notebook, especially words of encouragement or ideas. I flipped through this notebook and landed on this page.

Three truths about God:

1. God is perfect in love
2. God does what is best for us
3. Do not doubt him

OK, I thought, *"So God is infinite in his wisdom, he gives us direction, and he does not explain why".*

"But why would God give anyone cancer? So a cancer victim can share their story? Ha!" I thought skeptically, a smart-aleck thought; almost smirking.

In Rachel Remen's book *My Grandfather's Blessings*, she writes that "Curing is the work of experts, but strengthening the life in one another is the work of human beings." Let me expound on this author. She was a cancer doctor and in this book are short stories about her experiences treating cancer patients. Ultimately, that was exactly what my cancer doctor did for me. You will see as you read the next chapter. He was the expert who cured my cancer with surgery and radiation treatment. But, as a fellow human being, he also strengthened my life and soul. He was there for me to contact throughout the medical testing period, after my surgery, during my six weeks of radiation treatment, and in the several months after it, when tremendous fatigue plagued my body. But before I get into that too much, let me share with you a little more of my story. For the first time in my life of various medical treatments and care; <u>there was</u> a physician who cared about my wellness. It was this compassion from him that restored my faith in God and doubts about physicians' total commitment for wellness.

My faith in physicians' was greatly diminished when my youngest child was born. My pregnancy situation was the same as the stillbirth years before; she is here because my Obstetrician recognized problems in labor and performed a Cesarean section. The next morning after her birth, on his rounds at the hospital he explained that the cord was over the baby's shoulder and the baby was posterior (facing backwards); not allowing the baby to drop into the birth canal normally and a C-section was required. My face went white and he shockingly said to me; "You have lived through this before haven't you?" He was almost crying as he further stated, "Had I had any inkling of that; I would not have allowed you to become pregnant." This was like hearing baby Saul's birth situation again, same circumstances.

During an episode of Shingles my husband was treated with cortisone shots. Shortly within weeks, he developed diabetes extreme enough to be insulin-dependent. Diabetes may not have appeared had the physician been more cautious and taken a family history of diabetes. He did not. My research produced this bit of information: *If a direct family member has diabetes; avoid any cortisone medication as it can bring on diabetes in the next generation.* His maternal grandfather was diabetic.

Now to share my story.....

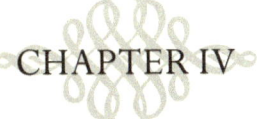

CHAPTER IV

My Story

(written for the KU ENT Department Grateful Patient Book)

M Y NAME IS JEAN M., and I am sixty-six years old. I use the "M" in my name, as Jean is such a common name. I like that the M can stand for "mother" or "me." I am a farmer's daughter, the oldest of four sisters with one older brother, an ex-wife of a farmer, and a senior human resources professional, now retired. I went out with flying colors by being named "Woman of the Year" for 2010–2011 in the industry of Medicare by the National Association of Professional Women. I had been working for the Centers for Medicare and Medicaid, U.S. government.

And now, I am a survivor of head cancer.

In May of 2010, after a one-day surgery, I received a biopsy report from Mayo Clinic that I had a rare tumor in my upper right nasal passage extending into my sinus cavities. As I tried to mentally absorb this life-threatening diagnosis, millions of questions popped into my mind. *Will I need more surgery? Will it require radiation or chemotherapy? Do I want to go through that? Do I refuse treatment and just go out into the world and live?*

I was told if I did the latter, the cancer would grow into my brain and right eye, resulting in blindness and death in a couple of years. My first reaction was denial and shock, along with hours of crying, *Why me?* I'd lost my firstborn child, a full-term baby, at birth many years ago, and felt I had already paid my debt to society. I immediately began reaching out to family, friends, and God.

I was either lucky, or it was a "God thing." I say that because my ear, nose, and throat specialist (ENT) in Lawrence, Kansas, Dr. Robert Dinswald, was very emphatic and supportive. He told me he would send me to one of the two best places for further treatment. The two possibilities were Kansas University Medical Center in Kansas City, Kansas, or Dallas Medical Hospital in Dallas, Texas. Dr. Dinswald referred me to Dallas Medical Hospital because that was where he received his training, but he initially set me up with an appointment for a second opinion with Dr. T. Grant of KUMC.

Before my first visit, Dr. Grant, had ordered lab tests, a PET scan, and a CT (CAT scan). By the time of this initial visit, I was exhausted, to say the least. During the consultation, he had access, via computer, to preliminary reports of the numerous tests. His resident physician examined my throat and neck. Dr. Grant examined my nasal passages. He was all business and did not converse much. He proceeded to set me up with appointments with a neurosurgeon and an eye surgeon. I guess I was still in shock, as I did not ask questions. When I think back, I know I was just numb to the world around me. Dr. Grant's nurse, Judy, gave me the date and time of my next appointment, which was to be on May 27, 2010.

The following Monday, Nurse Judy called to say they had scheduled my surgery for June 22. I was startled and stumbled out questions.

"Has Dr. T. Grant not talked to you about surgery?" she kindly asked.

I replied meekly, "No."

"I'll visit with him and call you back," she said.

The next evening, Dr. Grant called me and clarified why I needed surgery and further visits with specialists. He explained that he wanted to do this surgery before he left for a three-week vacation, and that the two-month window of opportunity for successful treatment would be closing if we waited till his return.

I told him that Dr. Dinswald, my first ENT, had wanted me to go to Dallas Medical Hospital if extensive surgery was required. Dr. Grant said that if I didn't trust him to do the surgery, he could get me an appointment with another ENT specialist for a third opinion.

"It wasn't that I do not trust you," I explained. "But I am being choosy and want the best; this is my head we are talking about."

He told me, that was why he wanted me to see a neurosurgeon and an eye surgeon, as the tumor might be growing into my brain or even into my right eye behind the orbital lining.

Dr. Grant was thorough in his explanations. He stated that he would do the surgery by going up the right nasal passage. If he saw the tumor growing into the brain, the neurosurgeon would do brain surgery right then. If the tumor was growing into the eye lining; he would have an eye surgeon standing by during the operation. He also told me that the PET scan (complete body scan) showed three other places in my body that alerted him, and he wanted to do more CT scans and MRIs to rule out another sarcoma somewhere else in my body. The "hot" spots showing on the PET scan; were in the right lung, the lower back, and the kidney area. He referred me to a hematologist in regard to the spot on my lung that had been diagnosed twelve years ago as a hamatoma (calcium deposit). He was concerned that the nasal sarcoma was not primary. I made numerous phone calls to have records, surgeries, x-rays, and MRI's sent to Dr. Grant of diagnoses of problems with the other hot spots and my other surgeries. I was amazed; he was on top of everything with such quick thinking and planning. He was making sure that this was the only tumor growing. Additionally, my family wanted me to go to KUMC because they would be close by. They too, were impressed by Dr. Grant's knowledge, his research into my case, and the treatment plan.

I went through two more visits with specialists and had additional MRI and CT scans before the June 22 surgery. Dr. Grant and the other specialists gave me very thorough exams and told me what to expect. Every doctor involved in my treatment was kept abreast of my case through an intricate computer network system; each physician viewed my tests and scans and added his notes. (Throughout it all, I kept saying I would write a book about this "long, hot summer that was," and it was a hot and long summer for me). My doctor team determined that the Para nasal sinus cavity was the primary site of my sarcoma. Thankfully, the other areas of concern in my body showed no signs of cancer. The day of my surgery essentially disappeared from my awareness, because the surgery lasted over seven hours. Dr. Grant was able to remove ninety-eight percent of the tumor; the rest was growing into my skull bone.

Dr. Grant consulted my daughters around 4:00 p.m., about six hours after my surgery started. Of course, my daughters were relieved to see him because of how long the surgery was taking. The doctor and my daughters discussed the portion that he said was in my skull bone. He discussed with them that the option for radiation seemed the best treatment at this point; possibly a need for six to seven weeks of radiation to arrest this cancerous portion growing into the bone. The girls agreed with Dr. Grant.

My care after surgery was awesome. The nurses and doctors frequently checked in on me during my two days of hospitalization. My radiation therapy, consisting of thirty treatments, began on August 2, 2010. My children discussed my having these treatments in Wichita, Kansas, because I would be closer to home and to one of my daughters to stay. But, Dr. Grant insisted that we at least go through a radiation evaluation at University of Kansas Cancer

Center, and I was grateful that we did. He also told me about Hope Lodge, a free, temporary residence provided by the American Cancer Society to patients receiving cancer treatment in another city. After my evaluation consultation, I was sold on getting treatments for radiation at KU Cancer Center. The chief oncologist, Dr. W. Chen, explained that this sarcoma tumor was in a delicate place that involved the optic nerve of my right eye and the pituitary gland. He told me that KU Cancer Center had the newest machine in the state.

After my first radiation treatment, I was referred to see Dr. Chen right afterward. I had consultations like this every Monday until my treatment was finished. I learned at my first visit that Dr. Grant had personally met with Dr. Chen to map the treatment area on my nose and between my eyebrows. They only used beams of intensity that my retina and optic nerve could tolerate in those sensitive areas; stronger beams were used at the point where the tumor grew into my skull bone. Dr. Chen had access to all scans, MRIs, and surgery notes, but Dr. Grant made doubly sure with the map that those beams were directed to the right areas. Any miscalculation could damage my right eye, causing loss of vision, or lead to pituitary gland impairment. A mask was molded to my face and shoulders, marking my eyes, nose, and mouth. To keep my head perfectly still during the radiation treatments, the mask was clamped to the table. Who could ask for better care from their cancer surgeon? Who could ask for more from their oncologist?

I have nothing but praise for Dr. Grant's skills and planning of my cancer treatment. He was there supporting me and cheering me on all the way through. Dr. W. Chen was there every week as well, checking on my progress and staying updated on any problems I had. I had two places of hair loss about two inches square and experienced some nausea toward end of treatments.

Now, six months later, I am working part-time for a small financial services company and slowly getting back into the swing of things.

I had resigned my job from the Centers for Medicare and Medicaid Services, US government, due to health reasons, and took retirement as I was at full retirement age. And, best of all, I can say,

"I am a cancer survivor! Praise God!"

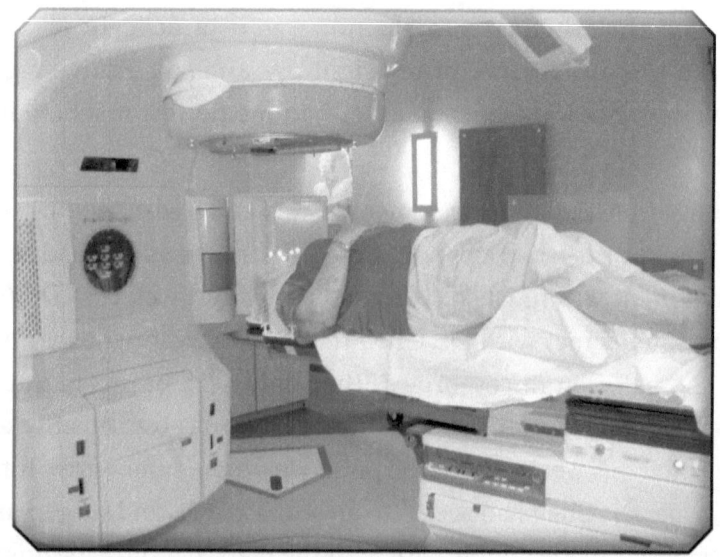

This is the Radiation machine at the Kansas University Cancer Center.

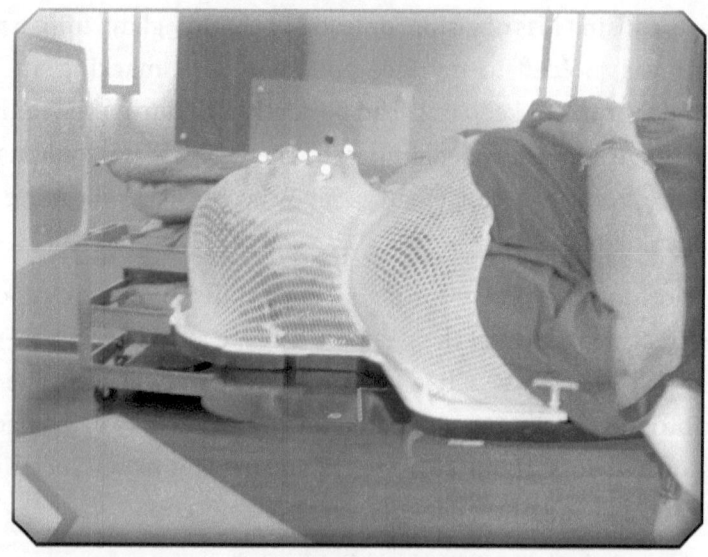

This is a picture of me during a treatment showing the mask that was used during all the radiation treatments.

CHAPTER V

Strengthening Others

"WHEN YOU STRENGTHEN THE life around you, perhaps you strengthen the life within you," from the book, *My Grandfather's Blessings* by Rachel Remen, MD.

So now when I go to Hope Lodge, I try to strengthen the lives around me. I stay there sometimes when I have a follow-up appointment. I spent six weeks living at Hope Lodge during my radiation treatment. Several of us lived there at the same time, and now we always touch base with each other through phone calls, text messages, or by visiting the lodge. Sometimes, someone is there for a follow-up visit like me. I know when you help others; one always has a 'feel good' feeling. You might say it 'strengthens the life' in yourself. Here again, I want to encourage and strengthen anyone reading this book by sharing these tips I came across in my Internet searches, book readings, and newsletters.

Tip 1.

"Journeying Together: Before and After Cancer Treatment"

This article I found in a newsletter, *Cancer Action* of Kansas City.

Professor of psychology David Greene, PhD, from the University of Saint Mary, gives interactive lectures with topics for patients actively undergoing treatment, their caregivers, and others. He states the following:

> Every relationship goes through its own rollercoaster of emotional ups and downs, but staying the course can be especially difficult when cancer is present. The emotional impact of a cancer diagnosis and treatment changes relationships continually, creating a new normal for the person living with cancer and the caregiver or partner. We all wear different roles and hats (husband, wife, caregiver, parent, patient, etc.) and need to learn how to navigate our relationships through this challenging time.

My own relationships with my children changed; in that they were the only people I wanted to be around. The desire to restore a relationship with my ex-husband was so strong; wanting the secure feeling of my former established home. Material things became irrelevant; all that mattered was the people in my life---those closest to me.

Tip 2.

"Coping with Cancer and Other Life Challenges," from Coping University Newsletter, Nov 2, 2010.

> How do you cope with cancer or another difficult life challenge? Here is a great idea to help you with coping, explained in a clip from "You Can Handle More Than You Think You Can," a presentation recorded live in front of one thousand oncology nurses. This popular program has earned rave reviews all over the country from patients, caregivers, nurses, and doctors. The presenter, Dave Balch, was caregiver for his wife

throughout her four bouts with breast cancer. She survived the cancer, and he survived taking care of her! In this DVD, he shares some of the coping strategies that helped them get through the ordeal, together, with love and humor. It is wonderfully entertaining, very funny, and touching, and it offers specific, practical things you can do immediately to reduce the stress and give you hope. In this clip, he talks about how important it is to have something to look forward to and shares how he and his wife used this technique to help get her through her chemotherapy. Visit www. HandleMore.com for more information about this DVD.

To prevent claustrophobia during my fifteen to twenty minute Radiation sessions, I prayed to keep my mind on something else. My oldest daughter, Lisa, encouraged me during those Radiation treatment weeks to plan a trip to Washington State to visit my youngest daughter, Malee, and family. And, I did so as I describe later in this writing.

Tip 3.

Getting Through the Shock of a Devastating Diagnosis

It could happen tomorrow. The doctor says, "I'm sorry, I have bad news..." and suddenly your life is turned upside down, leaving you reeling from the shock of a potentially life-threatening diagnosis.

Quoted by social psychologist Jessie Gruman, PhD, author of *AfterShock: What to Do When the Doctor Gives You—or Someone You Love—a Devastating Diagnosis*. She has been in this situation herself, *five times*, during her four separate bouts with different types of cancer plus the diagnosis of a dangerous heart condition. The following information is from this book:

Dr. Gruman suggests. *What helps...*

- **Treat the situation as a crisis.**

  It *is* a crisis—so consider what you need to do to take care of yourself right now and do *only* that for the first forty-eight to seventy-two hours. Call in sick instead of going to work...sleep in or nap if you can...cry when you feel like it...watch TV in bed...take a walk if you feel closed in or agitated...eat what you want, when you want (but be sure to eat *something*, even if you're not hungry, or you'll feel even more depleted). Give yourself this time to process what you've been told and start coming to terms with your situation. Remind yourself that you won't feel like this forever—as time goes on, the shock wears off.

- **Avoid making hasty decisions.**

  You may feel driven to start treatment immediately or have surgery *now* so you can put this problem behind you. But unless there is an actual emergency, it is better to slow down--because decisions made under duress are unlikely to be the best ones. There is rarely only one way to treat a disease, so take time to do some research, investigate your options, get a second opinion, and find the right specialist.

  "You do have to tread a careful path between rushing in and delaying treatment unnecessarily...but there is no time in your life when it's more important to make careful and informed decisions. The only thing you *must* accomplish during the first forty-eight hours is to set up appointments to see your doctor and perhaps get some tests, so you will know when you'll have more information upon which to base your decisions," Dr. Gruman said.

Just like Dr. Gruman said, ""Receiving bad health news sparks great personal upheaval...it is a time when nothing is certain and the future looks dark." In my situation, decisions were being made by me and my oldest daughter, as she was my Power of Attorney. I really relied on her as I was dealing with the initial shock still. I only had a two-month window for my treatment to be successful, decisions had to be made. I had to come to terms with my situation; even though I balked at the thought and did not want to hassle with making any decisions. Even thought of not going forward with any treatment; just live with it till death.

- **Try not to blame yourself.**

  Dr. Gruman points out. "Even if past behavior did influence your current health, the point now is not to blame yourself, but to make decisions that will help minimize the disease's impact going forward."

In my emotional upheaval, I blamed circumstances and others; more than blaming myself. I put a lot of blame on the stress in my life; from divorce; supporting myself for years; living with the mood swings of a Type I diabetic; family smokers; a high-stress job; etc. Stress destroying the immune system; letting a cancer grow. I did blame myself regarding the long hours of exposure to the direct sun; because I did have some control over that. I had to turn my negative feeling into positive energy. Feeling guilty did not change anything; did not make the cancer go away or erase the experiences of treatment from my mind. I had to learn to not use guilt as an excuse; but to use it to motivate myself.

- **Don't try to force yourself to be constantly optimistic.**
  In reality, hope is sometimes hard to hang onto, and it's perfectly normal to slide back and forth between despair and hope--even multiple times during a day. Dr. Gruman emphasizes, "Expressing fear, sadness or anger will not make your disease worse---remaining upbeat all the time

may prevent you from getting the support you need during this tough time."

This statement is so, so true. One swings back and forth between despair and hope; despair, 'I just want to forget---to be free from this'; despair, wanting to call daughters constantly for reassurance; hope, make a list of "to do's" for tomorrow; hope, 'pick a long wanted movie or book'; or hope, 'plan my calendar with visits to children'.

- **Seek support from loved ones—loved ones who validate your feelings.** Endless optimism is not only an impossible standard to hold yourself to; it is also a terrible burden for others to impose upon you. Dr. Gruman recalled a case in which, when a hospital chaplain asked a breast cancer patient how she was doing, the woman's husband replied for her, saying, "She's doing great, she's a trooper, she's going to be just fine!" And the wife said, "You always say that, but at night I'm scared, I'm lonely, and I don't have anyone to talk to about how I really feel."

- *Lesson:* Surround yourself with people who will listen to your honest concerns and who say, "I'm scared too, but I love you and I'm here for you," Dr. Gruman says.

If it wasn't for my long discussions via cell phone with my three children, I would not have made it through the diagnosis, the surgery, and mostly the months of fatigue and desperate lost feelings after Radiation and retirement; 2011 to early 2012. Taking Retirement came as a result of the diagnosis and full retirement age had hit at the same time, so it was a possible. It was a double whammy; to be at home (retired) every day and not receive the positive feedback from a daily job, and accepting my cancer situation at the same time.

Also, becoming involved in SPOHNC, a Head and Neck Cancer support group of Kansas City, after treatment gave me so much insight as to others' head or neck cancer survivorship experiences.

Tip 4.

This tip was taken from *Bottom Line* newsletter. Kristin Neff, PhD author of *Self-Compassion: Stop Beating Yourself Up and Leave Insecurity Behind* and associate professor in the educational psychology department at the University of Texas at Austin. She says:

"Our ultra-competitive culture tells us that we need to be constantly *above average* to feel good about ourselves —but there is always someone more successful, intelligent, or attractive than we are. And when we can't fool ourselves into believing that we're the best, we lose faith in ourselves and feel hopeless."

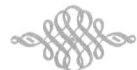

I spent many hours at Hope Lodge in Kansas City, courtesy of the American Cancer Society during my treatment. Other patients living there were seeking treatment from area hospitals for all kinds of cancer, from brain cancer to leukemia to bone cancer. We slowly became a close-knit group, and to this day we stay in contact with each other and give status updates. We have even had reunion dinners at Hope Lodge when some of us return for a short stay, either for further treatment or follow-up exams.

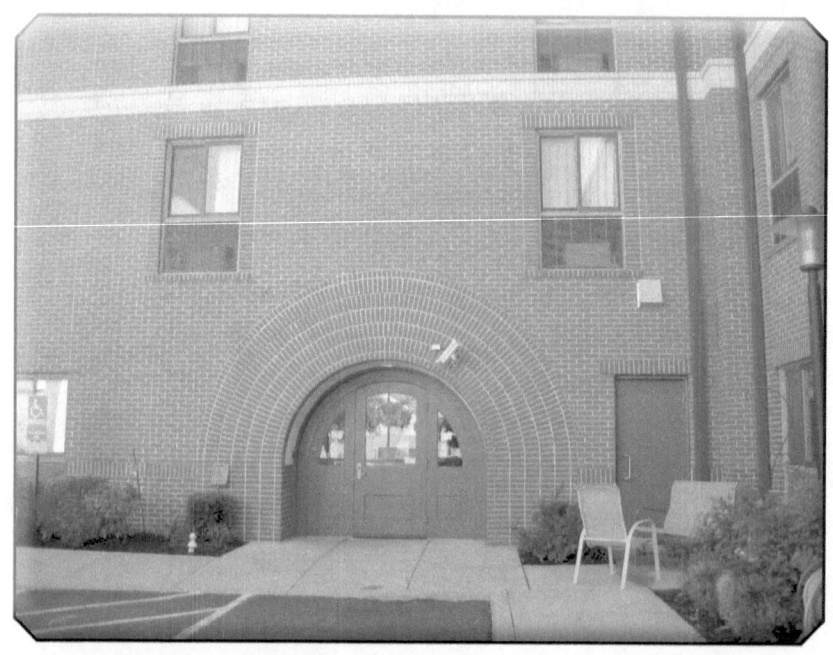

Hope Lodge a place for cancer patients to live; like a hotel.

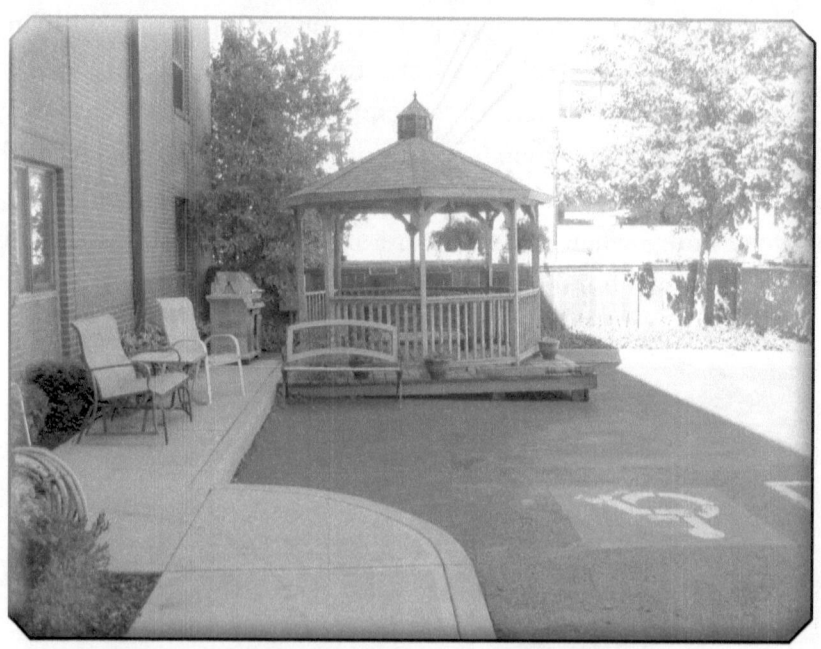

*Many hours of visiting with other cancer patients on the
back patio or in the gazebo of K.C. Hope Lodge.*

CHAPTER VI

Pay It Forward

To have something to look forward to during my treatment, my children encouraged me to plan a trip to Seattle, Washington area, where my youngest daughter and her family live and also my sister and her family, and Sequim, Washington, on the Olympic Peninsula, where first cousin Jerry has his retirement home.

Here is an essay I wrote to win a trip. I did not win the contest but will share this story for you.

Grandparents Day 2011 Contest Essay
by Jean Hadsell-Hahn Rusco

I found out what true grand-parenting was this past January and February. My youngest daughter Malee, age twenty-eight, packed up her and her children's few belongings overnight and left her marriage and a home where domestic violence had occurred. She was in fear for her life and the children's lives.

She moved in with a single girlfriend, who had three young children of her own, just three weeks before Christmas. She called me twenty days later and asked me to come help her; it was one thousand eight hundred (1,800) miles from my home in Kansas to Olympia, Washington.

I arrived January 1, 2011, and my daughter met me at Seattle–Tacoma airport. Her eight-year-old daughter and six-year-old son were with her. What a true joy for me as grandmother to see them and hold their hurting hearts.

My daughter's husband was very controlling, and she was not emotionally able to make any decisions. Her husband had threatened her life and put extreme fear in the children.

I was there filling in as mom, grandmother, and decision maker. I helped with groceries and food preparation for all eight of us in her girlfriend's home. Thank goodness she had a four-bedroom house with two baths. I again in my life became cook, laundress, and housekeeper, loving every minute helping those I so love. I even became a legal advisor and financial advisor.

Offering my support to my daughter and my grandchildren was exactly what we all needed—it helped me because it took my mind off my serious health issue. Just six months before, I had been diagnosed with a very rare, cancerous tumor in my nose and sinus cavities—a diagnosis followed by a lengthy surgery and radiation treatments.

This daughter and children had flown to Kansas City for my surgery, so this was my opportunity to show unconditional love by supporting them emotionally and spiritually.

After five long weeks of legal battles, my daughter finally received court-ordered full custody of the children and child support. Her spouse was given notice of a five-year restraining order. These last four months when she'd learned her spouse was cheating on her had been such a stressful time for her, but now she was seeing hope for the future. The hardest thing for her to deal with was the loss of her home and what used to be "family life."

It was, and is, my strongest desire for her and her children to relocate closer to Kansas, her home state and the place where her family lives. She planned on doing that, but not till after the children finished their school year in June 2011.

Now, six months later, she has met a wonderful man who treats her well and *normally*. She has turned to God and has been blessed with a new management job, which starts next week. At this point, she plans to stay in Washington.

One week after arriving in Washington, my pregnant oldest daughter (who lives south of Wichita, Kansas) gave birth two weeks early. It had been planned that I would be with her when she was dismissed for home so that I might help her care for the new infant during her first week with him. As it happened, I did not see my fourth grandchild till he was five weeks old, but he and his parents met me at the airport. Lots of cooing and kissing! Babies are so sweet.

To win this contest prize would be the greatest gift for me and three others—my daughter and my two grandchildren in Washington. Being a grandparent is the most wonderful joy, second only to the birth of one's own children.

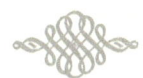

CHAPTER VII

Our Country Home

"**H**AVE YOU GOT A hold of your end of it? Be careful; these old steam pipes are hard to handle. We do not want to disturb the asbestos wrapping. There are nine more pipes to get out of this basement. My arms are really tired from using a hacksaw to cut these three-inch pipes over my head," my husband, Gene, told me. "After we get this pipe out and into the truck, we need to get some help to carry the old steam radiators out of the upstairs. I believe there are three big ones and one that is half-size," Gene said.

The pipes were three inches in diameter, wrapped in a thick waffle embossed asbestos paper. Because of age, it was flaking off in pieces; some pieces still hanging on the pipes. The house was built in 1913, and steam heat was the original heating system. The system had been replaced with a forced air gas furnace. At the time of this project, the house and the paper were sixty years old. Getting the radiators out from the upper story was an adventure. We hired a couple of strong boys from our hay crew to carry the smaller one out of the half bath and down the curved stairway. It was a tricky staircase. It was enclosed on both sides, and three steps down there was a tight curve. The spiral, wedge-shaped steps were wide on the outside of the curve and narrowed down to about two inches on the inside of the curve. Taking this radiator down one step at a time took almost thirty minutes. As big as our old country home was, the stairway was very narrow—it must've been where the owner-builder had cut corners on cost.

These solid cast-iron radiators were about three-and-a half-feet tall and about two-and-a-half-feet wide. The smallest one was about half that size in width only. The three others were in the bedrooms. We used our "think tank" to come up with a different method of getting the other three out of the house. At the top of the stairway, facing west, were two tall, four-foot-wide windows. We opened the northernmost window as wide as possible and moved the radiators out of the bedrooms and into the hallway. To describe the hallway the southern-most window was over the curved stairway; the northern window over the hallway floor where the steps ended. Using throw rugs to avoid damaging the windowsill, three men lifted each radiator to windowsill level and pushed it out the window as hard as possible so it would fall away from the house a few feet. This was about a twenty-five-foot drop. It was a day's project. From this point, the tractor was brought into play. With the tractor bale fork, my husband was able to chain the radiators, one at a time, to the hydraulic bale fork and lift each one onto the wheat truck bed along with the many pipes we'd removed. These were hauled a mile north to a pasture, where the lift on the wheat truck was put in gear; the cast iron debris pile slid out of the truck bed and onto the ground. (Years later, the pile was sold as scrap iron.) What a relief it was to have this project completed.

Our home was a beautiful bungalow home. All the floors were hardwood. The whole house had forty-nine windows. Six small dormer windows were set vertically into the north upstairs bedroom. These six windows, along with built-in solid pine window-seat cabinets under them for storage, stretched across the north side of the room.

The south bedroom had six much taller dormer windows and a short solid pine window-seat about 14" above the floor that spanned the entire south side of that room. Each bedroom had a large walk-in closet. The windows gave a spacious look and feel to each room, as one could see out for miles. Opening the windows during spring and fall allowed fresh air for sleeping.

For a country home, that many windows was not practical; central Kansas weather is windy and cold from the north during the winter, and hot, dusty winds prevail from the south in the summer. In the early years, the south bedroom on the main floor would have been used as a parlor. It had a large window on the south side of the house and an exterior door opened out onto a concrete and brick porch. On the west side were three sizeable windows. Those windows I covered with light green shantung draperies to keep out the cold and heat. The north-facing, main floor bedroom offered perhaps the most impractical use of windows—three large windows covered most of the north wall, and two large windows faced west. North rooms in Kansas receive the brunt of winter winds and snow. The living and dining area ran north to south and measured thirty-five feet by twenty feet; a hallway with oak colonnades separating the living space from the dining space. Each ceiling had decorative oak molding around the sides where the walls met the ceiling.

The homestead owner, himself, built a walnut buffet on the north end of the dining room; it measured about eight feet by two feet. It had six small drawers in the center and glass double doors covering the shelves on either side of the drawers. Old-fashioned glass knobs adorned the doors and drawers. There were four short windows (two sets) across the north wall above the built-in buffet. My decorator created a continuous color effect by making gold silk, sheer curtains, shirred on rods at both the top and bottom. This way, these windows could be opened in the warmer months for better airflow, yet, the attached curtains wouldn't fly in the breeze and, at the same time, let in lots of light.

There was a built-in oak roll-top desk in the hall between the east colonnades. A redbrick fireplace was situated diagonally on the living room side of this desk & hall. The colonnades on the west side of the living-dining areas led to the back hallway, where the bedrooms, bathroom, and stairway were situated. The bathroom had the original fixtures and period terrazzo floor tile. The whole house had the original light fixtures. In the full basement was a shelf for the large batteries used for power before electricity.

Over the years we did so much to that house, fixing it up from lack of upkeep over the years, and updating some features. We put new storm windows and screens on all forty-nine windows and installed a sliding door that led from the enclosed porch to the outside porch, along with four new storm doors. Two of the storm doors at the front of the house were decorative— amber glass panels and brown aluminum. We painted the trim on windows and eaves to match the brown of these doors, and eventually replaced the antiquated green shingles.

For that job, we hired our hay harvesting crew and did the re-shingle project ourselves in matching brown. The outside of the house was beige stucco over red tile blocks. These blocks expanded and contracted with temperature changes. The dining room walls would crack each year at the point where the inside portion met the outside wall; about four feet in.

It was an estate home with land totaling 360 acres. My husband came out of the Navy in 1970, and we made the purchase in March 1974. Our son was one year old at the time. We purchased the land and home from the daughter of the man who homesteaded the property and built the home. She'd inherited the home and land, which also included a small barn and raised her family in the home. When I say "homesteaded," I'm referring to the process of building a home on a tract of land, with the intent to live there and farm. The south quarter (160 acres) was homesteaded by planting forty acres of trees called "timber claim" In order to acquire the land from the government at a minimal price, many tracts of land had some acreage in trees which were planted by the homesteader to claim the land.

The large kitchen was where I spent my time. We removed the heavy oak swinging door between it and the dining room to improve the heating in the kitchen. The room was twenty feet by fifteen feet with a laundry area located on the north end and entry to basement stairway and a garage. Birch cabinets extended from floor to ceiling on the east wall, and an island that housed the stove divided the room. An exterior door opened onto an enclosed porch. All the doors leading outside were heavy oak doors with beveled glass panes. The parlor had two oak French doors to the living room, also with beveled glass panes.

This kitchen had a built-in ironing board, which was very common in homes built during that era. Even though it was old-fashioned, I loved it. The ironing board was easy to get out for a quick press and easy to put away out of sight—it was housed behind a small door in a wall cavity. As we have progressed into the 2000s, most clothing does not require ironing or a great deal of care anymore, but during our early years there I was a seamstress, making clothes and sleepwear for our young children. I was very frugal because I knew how hard my husband worked to provide for us.

The extra wide chimney at the back of the fireplace was the southwest wall of the kitchen. The heat made the plaster crackle, and we knew that paint or wallpaper would not last there, so we covered the wall with square cork tiles. This idea turned out to be the best thing we could have done. On this cork wall we displayed family pictures, schoolwork, art made by our kids, ribbons and awards.

On the south wall were three windows looking out to the enclosed porch. Orange burlap fabric valances were made to tie in with the country look. A wooden rod halfway up the windows had orange curtains to give our kitchen dining area privacy, when company came to the kitchen door. This was an everyday occurrence with farmers as neighbors to come to the back door. Above the kitchen sink on the east side, two small windows offered a view of the pasture to the draw, with cottonwood trees.

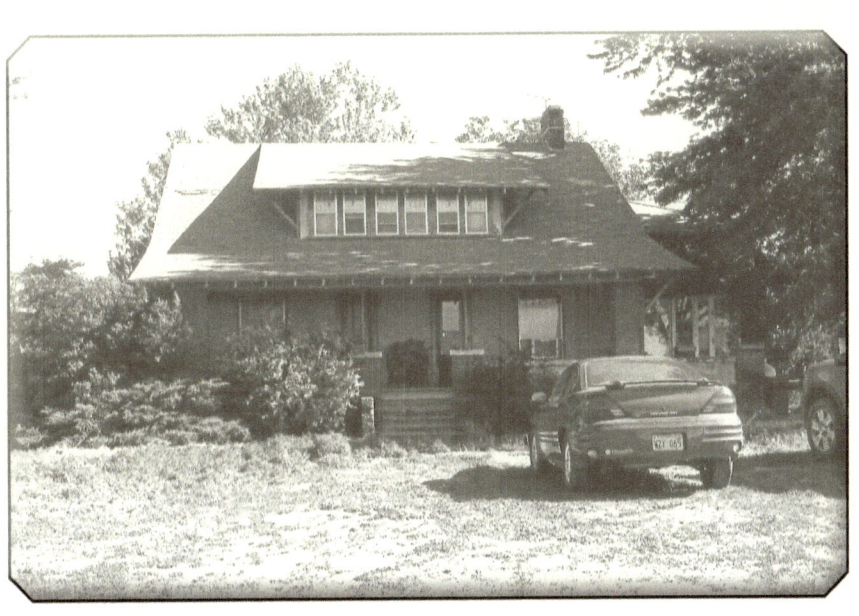

CHAPTER VIII

Our Farming Operation

THIS DRAW—A WATERWAY WHEN it rained—ran across the east side of the property a half mile away. The draw, or dry creek, came across our 360 acres at the half-mile line south of our house and divided the land in two tracts. When it reached the east side of the property, it went straight north to the road ditch. My husband had cleared the trees from the draw that divided the land into two halves (each half called a quarter section of land). The draw only had water after rains or snowmelts. He did this to avoid the inconvenience of dragging his equipment around the trees. (To better envision the lay of the land, take note of the background in the picture on the front cover.)

For nine years, my husband, Gene, ran a custom haying operation. He designed a machine to pick up hay bales—we called it the "Green Monster." Many times he sold the customer's hay crop to buyers to be shipped via semitrailer to other states such as Missouri, Arkansas, Oklahoma, and Texas. Our "Green Monster" loaded these semi-trucks with hay. From April to October, we used a crew of four strong high school boys for the hay season; three would stack the hay on the machine with my husband as driver. Then the machine would be driven to the designated place to stack the hay and the three men would stack the hay on the ground making a 20-25' tall by 15' wide hay stack or stack in a shed. The "Green Monster" had a conveyor system that pulled the bales in the field up to the machine bed, till stacked 3 high and 5 wide. Then the conveyor carried the bales down to be stacked.

The fourth young man would operate the equipment to prepare the land for planting. This person had to be a trusted, responsible individual, as heavy equipment, such as tractors and hay balers can be dangerous to operate if they did not follow Gene's operating instructions. It was hot, dusty work and if the hay had been rained on, it had to sit several days to dry out, and would become moldy. Breathing this dry mold dust can be an environmental hazard; believe me, my husband and myself were in direct contact with it many times.

We were dry land farming, wheat, alfalfa hay, feed, and oats. One of our neighbors irrigated the half section west of us, and another neighbor had a quarter to the north and a quarter to the east of our land under circle irrigation. When there is circle irrigation, fertilizer, insecticides, and pesticides—and sometimes weed and grass pre-emergence—are added to the water and sprayed through large sprinklers about seventeen feet above the ground onto the land. Of course, with our Kansas winds, we received the drift from these circles of water. These irrigation farmers also had chemicals sprayed by airplane, and the planes always flew over our farm homestead, ending the spray at the end of our driveway and turning back over our house. I know we received lots of drift with the overhead spraying because the planes dropped a strip of white paper when the spray was shut off, and I would find many of these strips on our property. I can clearly remember making my children come inside when aerial spraying was in process, just to be on the safe side. But had that been enough to protect us? Breathing these chemicals from irrigation and aerial spraying is very dangerous to a person's long range health.

CHAPTER IX

Possible Causes

"**L**OGIC CAN BRING SMARTS; imagination can create a life of possibilities." As a cancer survivor, I can say that it helped me to post this motto everywhere to get through the fatigue and depression caused by treatment. Another helpful post is Jeremiah 29:11.

> "For I know the plans I have for you," declares the Lord, "plans to prosper you and not harm you, plans to give you hope and a future."

What caused my cancer? This question nagged at me for months after surgery and all during the six weeks of Radiation, and it still haunts me. I did research to find out my expected life span after treatment, and the research articles state up to five years for an individual with sarcoma tumor. Two years have passed, and I am still writing. How much longer do I have? I do wonder. My research revealed that the overall five-year relative survival rate combining all stages and types of sarcoma; is approximately, fifty-one percent.

However, when the sarcoma is located in an arm or leg, the five-year survival rates are slightly higher for each stage. How long a person lives with sarcoma depends on many factors, including the size of the tumor, where it is located, the type, the mitotic rate (how fast the tumor cells are growing and dividing), and whether it is superficial or deep (stage). If the sarcoma is diagnosed at an early stage and hasn't spread from where it started, treatment is very effective and many people can be cured. Thank goodness my tumor had not spread.

The physicians told me that my tumor had been growing for some time, possibly four or five years. I was asked when I noticed changes. I recalled a very serious sinus infection in the fall of 2004; at the time, I spent two weeks sleeping in my lounge chair in the upright position so I could breathe. My physician back then had prescribed an antibiotic and a decongestant, Claritin. Finally, after almost two weeks of no relief from severe sinus headaches, I called my daughter to take me to the emergency room. I was really afraid that the infection was putting me close to death; recalling a friend, years earlier, had passed away due to a severe sinus infection. My daughter suggested I quit the Claritin and take Sudafed instead. I followed her advice, and in one day I felt so much better. I was fearful of taking Sudafed, as it was and still is not recommended for a person taking high blood pressure medication like myself, but I could not believe how quickly I recovered and was back to feeling good and breathing well again. I think I was allergic to the decongestant.

Sometime after that, I started having symptoms of nasal allergies. I assumed it was the high mold count, which is always reported on the local weather reports for eastern Kansas. I purchased several different brands of allergy relief medications till I felt they were no longer working. I spent so much money on these products, I felt I was the only one keeping their makers in business.

What caused this strange type of cancer in my nose and sinus cavities?

Was it the fifteen years of secondhand smoke from my husband's habit?

At the beginning of my first pregnancy, I had begged my husband to quit, not wanting the baby to be exposed to smoke. His family would visit, and they all smoked in our home, too. It was not my preference; I have never been a smoker.

Was it the chemicals I was exposed to from the circle irrigation around our land and home or the aerial spraying of planes making their U-turns over our house?

Was it the exposure to asbestos-wrapped steam pipes? The small amount of time I handled them when carried the pipes out of our home thirty-five years ago.

Was it a floating sarcoma cell from the breathing-tube used during gallbladder surgery in 2008? I ask myself this question, because Dr. Grant explained to me that a sarcoma cell can be present in your bloodstream two days or twenty years and whenever it settles somewhere; it will grow another tumor.

Did it grow on my face due to excessive exposure to sunlight? I was a lifeguard for a city swimming pool for two years to help pay for my college. I also spent hours in the hot sun during wheat harvests.

Could it have been caused from living in cities with heavy smog? We lived in the San Francisco Bay area for eight months and the Los Angeles area for two years, both places having high levels of smog on a daily basis. This was time spent with my husband, who was stationed near these places during the Navy.

Was it the excessive amount of dust and chaff I inhaled? Wheat harvests—first as a teenager and later as a wheat farmer's wife of twenty years. Or could it be the moldy hay dust I breathed during hay season.

Could the exposure to numerous dust storms, during my youth, have caused this cancer to grow later in life?

CHAPTER X

Uncovering Childhood Experiences

A HA! THINKING BACK TO my early childhood, I remember my brother and I climbing up about twelve rungs on the side of the big Quonset building at our farm in western Kansas; we were about eight and ten years of age.

We grabbed the rope sack swing that Dad had rigged from the ceiling. Our wheat harvest of grain was piled in the center of the shed because the elevators were full.

So guess what we two farm kids dreamed up? To climb the side of the building, grab the sack swing, and hold on for dear life by clasping our knees over the sack. We would push ourselves off the side of the shed and swing over the pile of wheat, then let go for a big drop into the pile of grain, which spread like sand. What great fun it was! We had a laughing good time all afternoon, swinging and jumping into the pile of wheat repeatedly. We did not even notice that the pile became shorter and wider with each jump. At the end of the day, we received a long tongue-lashing from our father, and the sack swing was tied out of our reach.

Cattle and chicken feed was always packed in large burlap bags. The sack swing was one of these burlap bags stuffed with scraps of other bags to make a ball of burlap about the size of a basketball.

I remember that other burlap bags were used to wrap a ceramic water jug, which my father would take to the field with him for the day. This jug had a chain with a cork stopper attached to it. My father would fill his burlap-wrapped jug everyday with cool well water and soak the wrapped burlap on the outside of the jug in the stock tank, then tie the jug in front of the truck's radiator. The air passing over the wet burlap during the drive to the field kept the jug of water cool for most of the day.

I could write forever about my childhood in western Kansas as a farmer's daughter. I recall experiencing really bad dust storms when I was very young. We moved from central Kansas to western Kansas, twenty-six miles northwest of Tribune, Kansas. Our farm site was one mile from the Colorado line. The farmstead had a house, a windmill, an outhouse, and a small silver-colored tin barn. I remember our nightly ritual of mother taking us—my brother and me—to the outhouse before bedtime. My father was very ingenious. Within three months, he had finished the indoor bathroom, which even had running water.

There was no rural electricity in the late 1940s. I was about three years old when we moved, my older brother was about five, and my younger sister was a baby. My father purchased a generator, finished wiring our house, and powered electricity from the generator. The windmill and well were on a small hill across the driveway, east of the house. Father acquired a large enclosed water tank and mounted it on stilts beside the well. This allowed the water to flow downward toward the house. He buried the large water pipe under the ground across the sandy, rocky driveway to the full basement of the house. The house was not very old; it had two bedrooms, a living room, a dining room, a kitchen, and a large pantry that also housed the stairway to the basement. The house was finished on the main floor, except for the bathroom that Dad put in (sink, tub, and toilet; he also built the cabinets and a clothes-shoot to the basement laundry area.

My father did awesome things to that place in the eight years we lived there. He built a two-car garage, a large Quonset shed with a concrete floor, a long chicken house, and a brooder house on skids for starting baby chicks.

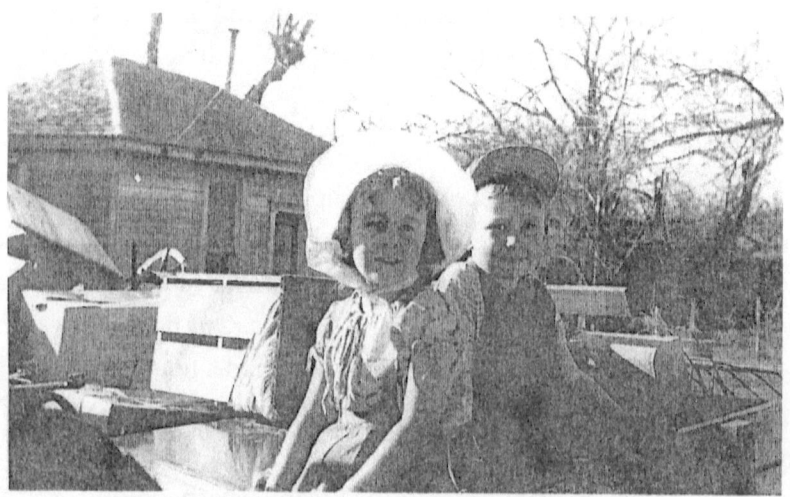

My brother and I sitting in the truck bed on Moving Day to Western Kansas.

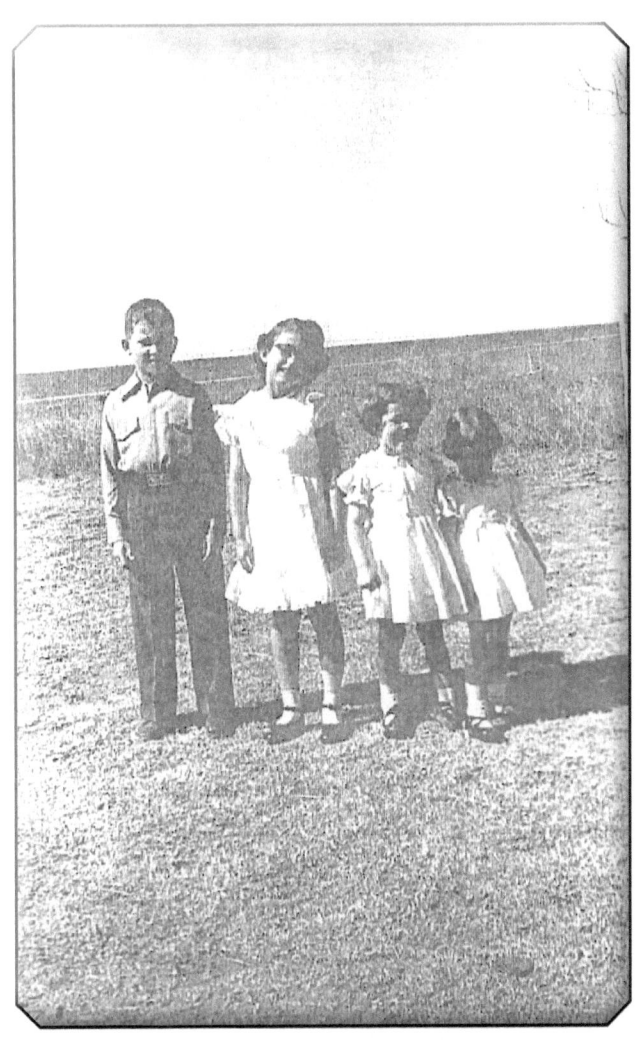

Brother, me, and two younger sisters, Easter
Sunday in Western Kansas, 1954 or 1955.

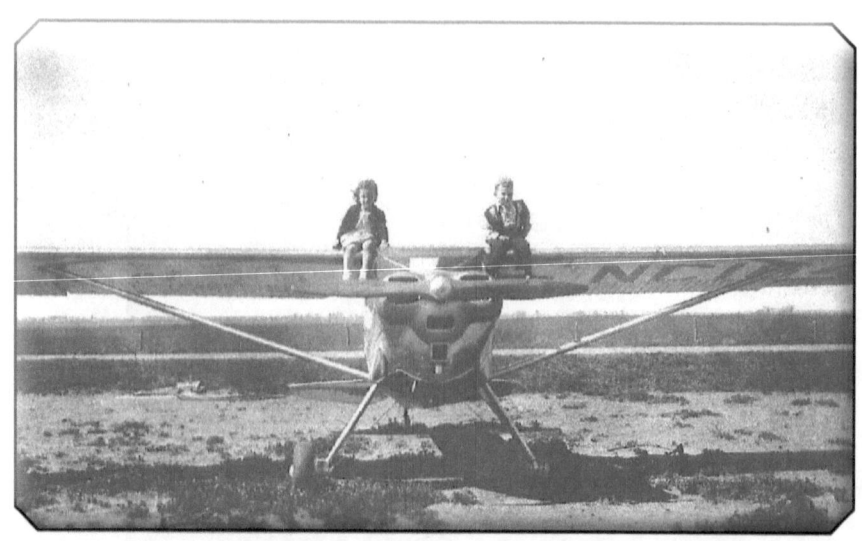

*Older brother, Dan and myself on wings of my father's
Cessna airplane on Western Kansas farm.*

The dust storms...I remember the worst one so vividly, like it was yesterday. I can still see the ominous cloud of black and brown swirling dust coming right at us. My brother and I had a chore after school each day—walk the pasture to bring in our two milk cows to the barn for the evening. Sometimes the cows were at the far end of the pasture, a half-mile away. On the day of this horrible storm, we began our walk north to get the cows; they were about three-fourths of the way to the end of the pasture. Finally, we reached them and got them turned toward the barn and farmstead. Starting back south, we were alarmed to see the huge cloud of dirt rolling toward us. The sky was black, like it gets during a severe thunderstorm, with brown dirt rolling and heaving about halfway up the sky, visible against the blackness of the storm. The dust covered the entire southwestern sky, making it become extremely dark early. We began running the cows to get back to the barn as quickly as possible. We were scared, and as the air turned chilly we finally reached the barn and corralled the cows through the door, shutting them inside. The wind hit fiercely, bringing with it flying dirt and sand from the driveway that stung our faces.

My mother and younger sister were trying to chase the two hundred young pullet chickens into the chicken house. We joined them in the fight to chase and shoo the young chickens, who were almost ready for butcher, toward the openings of the chicken house. If we didn't get them in out of the storm, they would likely smother. The dirt and wind became so thick and strong we could hardly see, let alone stand up steady against the furious wind. Mother finally yelled to us, "Grab each other's hands so none of you gets lost in this blinding dirt! I'll guide us to the house!" She continued, and we slowly worked in a line toward the house, bucking the wind and shielding our eyes against the stinging dirt and sand. The entire time mother yelled for us to hold on tight and continued talking so we could more easily follow her direction by her voice, since we could barely see her or each other. Dad had not come home yet from working a field several miles away, and he did not arrive home for some time. When we finally closed the house door behind us, we were shaking from the fear of getting lost in the dense fog of dirt. Mother hugged us all and quietly said that we should grab our bed pillows and a jackets and head for the basement. We will want them in case the electricity goes out from the high winds." We had rural electric power by now. Mother grabbed water-soaked towels and followed us down the stairs. She tacked the towels up against the south and west windows to keep the dust from filtering into the basement air. Before a towel went up, I looked out a west window; red dirt swirled against the glass so thick we could not see the other side of the concrete window well. The red dirt had to come from Oklahoma; Kansas dirt is gray-brown.

During another bad dust storm, my father got us lost. We had attended a grade-school program that my brother and I were in at our small country school about six miles from our farm home. Stinging sand struck our faces as we ran to our car. As Dad drove us home, the blinding dirt was so thick it was like a blizzard—only this was a blinding dirt storm. About halfway home on a country road with deep ditches, there was a T-junction, a three-way intersection connecting a northbound road with an east and west road. Dad and mom could only see the right side of the road as a guide. Mom soon realized they had unknowingly followed the curve because the dirt was swirling around the car, limiting visibility. My Dad too realized about a mile north of the junction that he was going the wrong way. He turned the car around and we finally made it home, creeping slowly at a snail's pace watching for clumps of dirt along the side of the road or wild sunflowers growing. to be sure we were on the road and not heading for the deep ditch.

If there was a dust storm while we were in school and someone needed to use the restroom, we had to go to the outhouse in pairs. I always hoped the teacher would not assign me to take another student, because I was deathly afraid of these storms after my experiences. By my second grade all the parents volunteered to install a bathroom inside the schoolhouse.

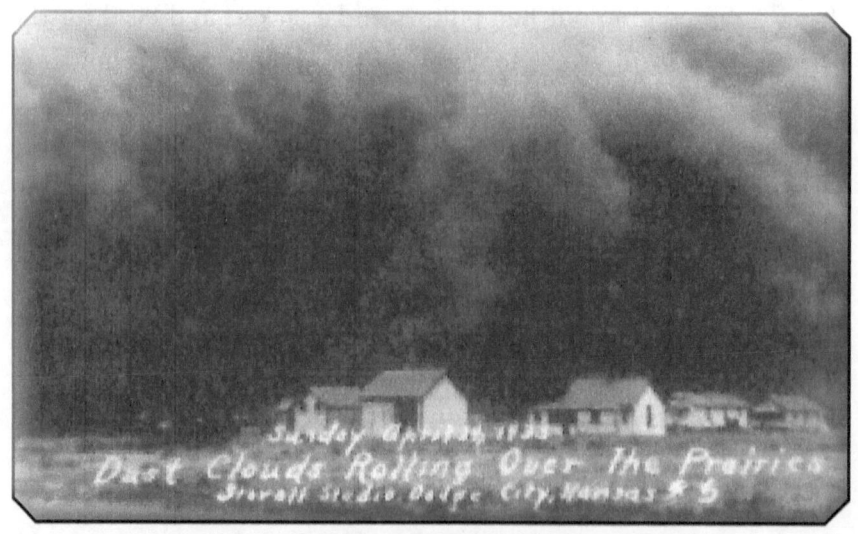

Dust storm looks very similar to the one we experienced, in the 1950's of Western Kansas.

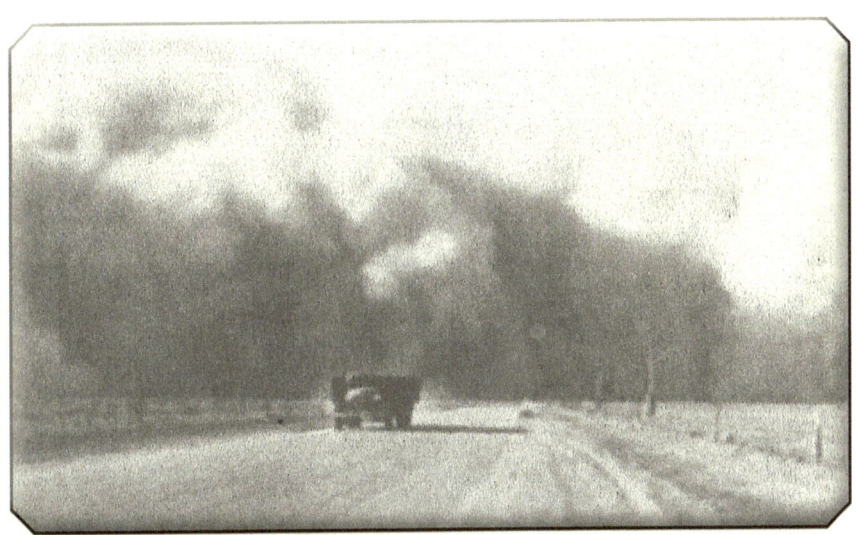

Looks like a loaded grain truck racing for cover to beat the dust storm. The fierce winds would blow large amounts of grain out of the truck.

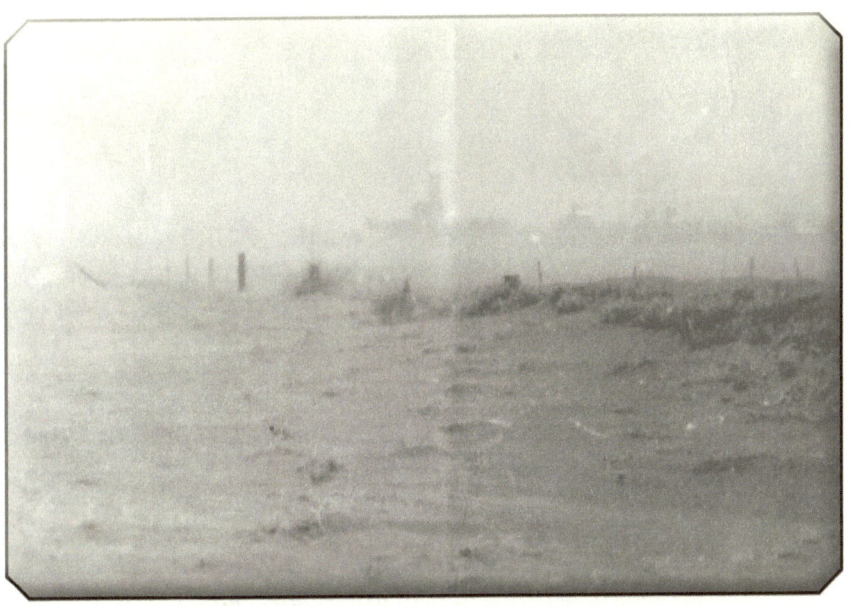

Fence row filled with dirt and sand after a bad dust storm. Note machinery buried, 1930's photo.

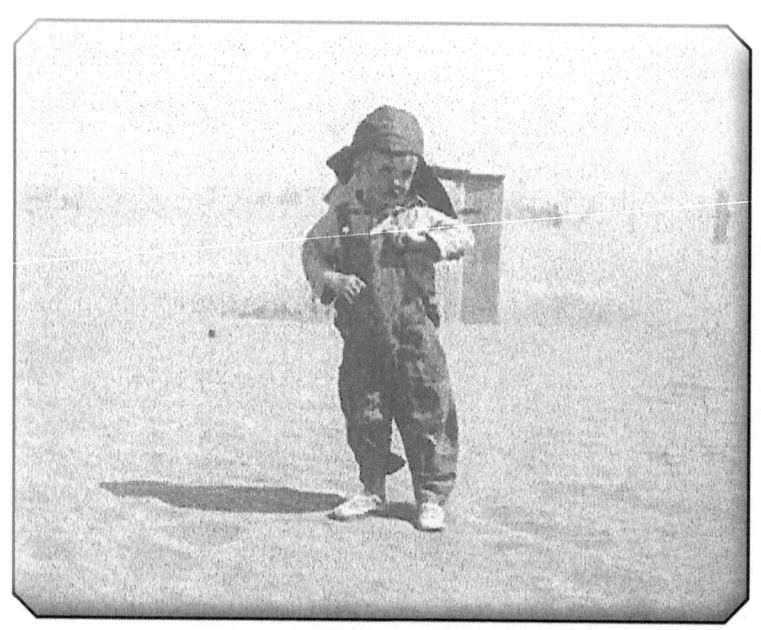

*This is what it looked and felt like on the runs
to the schoolhouse out house.*

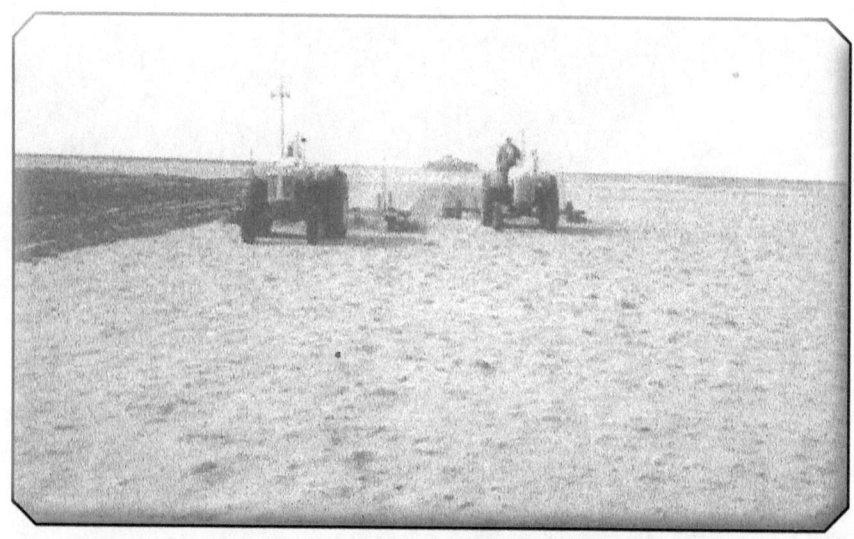

*Two farmers here tilling the soil using chisel shanks set 6-8
inches deep to stop the soil from blowing during the 1950's
drought. I can so vividly remember my father, frantically
turning the soil even during the blinding dirt.*

CHAPTER XI

The Silent Disease

MY MOST MEMORABLE FACE and nose pain was when the breathing tube was removed from my right nostril after surgery in early 2008. Thinking back, this could have been an indication that something was not normal with my right nasal passage. While in Dallas visiting friends in late 2007, I became very sick. After five hours of stomach pain and retching, I called the health clinic. I told the nurse I was coming in. After she had me describe my symptoms, she advised me to go immediately to the emergency room of Medical Center of Dallas hospital. I was not familiar with the area and had to ask for directions to the hospital. I managed to get myself into my car and took the freeway for seven miles to the large Dallas hospital emergency room. Finally, after hours of testing, a sonogram granted the diagnosis of a gallbladder attack. By that time, it was midnight, and I was medicated to relieve symptoms and kept overnight. The following morning a surgeon discussed having Laparoscopic surgery scheduled as soon as possible.

I remember waking up to see a blur of cloth curtains around me. Shortly, I became aware that I was in a recovery room after surgery. I was then taken to a hospital room. My surgeon, on his rounds, the next morning told me the organ was swollen very large and major surgery had to be performed. He told me that the anesthetist would come in and take out the breathing tube in my nose.

When the anesthetist appeared, I asked him, "Will this hurt?"

"Not bad," he replied. "Just hold the side of the bed, and I will take it out with a quick pull."

"Oh! Ow-w-w-w-!" I screamed. It felt as if he was pulling my nose off my face.

"I am surprised it was that painful," he said, puzzled. Not long after, the pain was gone. But now I wonder—*was the tumor growing in there at that time?*

"The more faithfully you listen to the voice within you, the better you hear," quoted by Dag Hammarskjöld, so, so true.

When it comes to personal health, a person has to be his or her own advocate—in other words, listen to the voice inside you and follow your gut instincts. I have often heard the comment, "Listen to what your body is telling you." I have learned that "the gut instinct" is God talking. These gut instincts I recognize as weird, uneasy feelings, as if things are not right. Even something like knowing you are going to hear unanticipated bad news; like a family tragedy—*the calm before the storm.*

There is something called the silent disease—a disease that is not diagnosed right away because it produces no obvious signs or symptoms. I was diagnosed with sleep apnea not that many years ago. How did that come about, you ask? My daughter, Lisa, complained of my catching my breath at night while snoring. If she hadn't done that, I might never have known I had a problem. I had spent the night at their home.

After testing, I received a diagnosis of sleep apnea in late summer of 2009. I asked the sleep doctor, "Could there be an obstruction in my throat, nose, or esophagus?" Her reply was, "It is very, very rare. You can seek out a specialist if you want, but you will be on this C-PAP machine the rest of your life."

After four months of using a C-PAP machine to sleep, with much frustration, I took the initiative to make an appointment with an otolaryngologist. As a direct result my of listening to my voice and taking action, I was diagnosed with polyps in my right nasal passage that extended into sinus cavities and later turned out to be a cancerous tumor there and beginning to grow into my skull bone.

Please talk to your doctor. Confront him or her if you are diagnosed with sleep apnea. If your doctor prescribes for you to use a C-PAP machine to increase oxygen in your system, ask him for a referral to an otolaryngologist for a second opinion.

I am a survivor due to my diligence and determination. I would like to see, as a standard; physician's make an automatic referral to an otolaryngologist for patients newly diagnosed with sleep apnea. "I know firsthand that this precaution saves lives—it certainly saved mine."

Other silent diseases can be misdiagnosed or symptoms noticed later after onset. Some of those diseases are, of course, cancer, diabetes, ALS, heart conditions, irregular blood pressure to mention a few.

CHAPTER XII

A Survivor

Now that I am a survivor, I am learning the challenges that come with being a survivor. Once the cancer is irradiated, we think that our lives will go on unchanged, but as we talk in our support groups, we find that not to be true.

Having been so well taken care of by my medical team, Hope Lodge, and my supporters, I quickly began asking for donations to the American Cancer Society for the Kansas City Hope Lodge to be able to purchase "cheery" shower curtains. I managed to gather six hundred dollars for this project. The previous shower curtains were white plastic and made visitors feel as if they were in a hospital shower. Now, Kansas City Hope Lodge has pretty and colorful shower curtains. This experience of doing something for cancer patients is not unusual, but it is rewarding.

Sometimes, I feel that my status as a survivor is not well received by other cancer patients who are having a harder time, by caregivers or family members who have lost a loved one to cancer. I see people involved in life-and-death cancer fights all the time, and they have been through much more than I have. I feel guilty sometimes because my type of cancer would not respond to chemotherapy, so I didn't have to go through that experience. At the same time, I am so thankful for that blessing. The challenge of chemotherapy is extreme, usually making one very ill, and it is associated with many unpleasant side effects.

As stated by David Hinz, a cancer survivor who wrote about his journey in a book called *My Private Mountain*, a culmination of like minds with experiences to share:

"What I have learned about the human spirit through my experiences with cancer is that the disease knows no bounds. Through our personal challenges, failures, successes, anger, love, spirituality, and so forth, we form a brotherhood; as survivors, we come together to make a difference so that others may not have to endure what we have."

I do not wish what my family and I have been through, on anyone. My struggle with cancer has opened me up to doing whatever I can on this earth to make life better for others in the future. Take the time to look inside yourself and share your life with others, and, above all, take in the beauty that exists around you. Take time to reflect or feel good about what you have done in your life. Don't focus on things you feel you did wrong. Rather, take time every day to think only about what you did right. No one is perfect; we all know that. At the end of each day write down a list all you did to care for your recovery and continued health. Focus on the positives to help inspire you to keep working on your goals.

Ask yourself what you tried and how it worked; think of what you learned. If something worked, ask yourself, 'why?' and if it did not work, ask yourself, 'what got in the way? and 'what you might do differently tomorrow?'. Focus on what you **can do** tomorrow.

Choose one thing at a time, that you know that you can accomplish. Don't try to do several things. A good place to start is with your biggest struggle or the thing that causes you the most stress. Then, take another step toward your goal every few days.

Taking care of your health after cancer is hard work; but it influences how you feel about yourself. Eating a healthy diet, choosing the right foods, exercising each day, getting enough sleep, gaining support are all regimens, we, as survivors have to keep focused on. For the support, find someone or a support group who can give you encouragement and cheer you on. Just sharing with others is tremendous loving support. Take time to reward yourself; after all, you made the efforts. Pat yourself on the back for all you have done, and all you do. You have definitely earned it!

Humble beginnings often find their way down unexpected paths toward unimaginable destinations. At this writing, the KU website features an article by Alissa Poh, *Solving the riddle of sarcomas through collaboration.* Excerpts from that article are as follows:

> The University of Kansas Cancer Center, which just received National Cancer Institute designation, July 12, 2012, is developing one such circular collaboration where ideas and observations cycle freely between clinicians and basic scientists. The aim: demystifying sarcomas, rare solid tumors of the body's tougher tissues such as muscles, nerves and bones. It's modeled after The Learning Collaborative (TLC), a public-private partnership between KU Cancer Center, the Leukemia and Lymphoma Society and the National Center for Advancing Translational Sciences (NCATS). For now, this new venture is simply known as the Sarcoma Learning Collaborative. Its genesis lies in the inevitable "How can we make a difference?" question that accompanies every cancer diagnosis

but is especially poignant when tackling rare forms of the disease, including sarcomas.

"From a drug development perspective, sarcomas are rare enough that pharmaceutical companies can't afford to spend much effort on them," says Scott Weir, Pharm.D., Ph.D., director of KU's Institute for Advancing Medical Innovation (IAMI) and one of TLC's founders. "By applying TLC's partnership model to sarcoma research, we've enabled multiple people to work together and address this unmet medical need." They hope to dramatically accelerate the pace at which better therapies against sarcomas are discovered and propelled to the clinic.

It is my desire that this book encourages others and gives them hope and strength. "...but strengthening the life in one another is the work of human beings." says Rachel Remen, M.D. I want to leave you with an article I found in my mother's things several years after her death:

PROMISE YOURSELF

Promise yourself to be so strong that nothing can disturb your peace of mind. To talk health, happiness, and prosperity to every person you meet. To make all your friends feel that there is something in them. To look at the sunny side of everything and make your optimism come true.

To think only of the best, to work only for the best and only of the best, and expect only the best. To be just as enthusiastic about the success of others as you are about your own. To forget the mistakes of the past and press on to the greater achievements of the future.

To wear a cheerful countenance at all times and give every living creature you meet a smile. To give so much time to the improvement of yourself that you have no time to criticize others. To be too large for worry, too noble for anger, too strong for fear and too happy to permit the presence of trouble. -Author unknown

My wish for you is to always love, bless, live, and follow your passion.

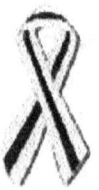

"The awareness ribbon is reprinted with the permission of SPOHNC(Support for People with Oral and Head and Neck Cancer) at www.spohnc.org. SPOHNC is dedicated to raising awareness and meeting the needs of oral and head and neck cancer patients."

www.ingramcontent.com/pod-product-compliance
Lightning Source LLC
Chambersburg PA
CBHW021254280526
45784CB00005B/2373